This Journal Belongs To:

____

Date________________________

Time	Fruits	Vegetables	Herbs/ Glandulars
	Raw/Whole? Frozen? Juiced? Smoothied?		Tea? Capsules? Raw/Whole? Dried?
05:00			
06:00			
07:00			
08:00			
09:00			
10:00			
11:00			
12:00			
13:00			
14:00			
15:00			
16:00			
17:00			
18:00			
19:00			
18:00			
19:00			
20:00			
21:00			
22:00			
23:00			

E.g. Rebounder, Inversion, High Jumps, Sauna

Slept or Fasted	Amount of Water Consumed	Sun Exposure	Lymph Exercises

Date________________________

Time	Fruits	Vegetables	Herbs/ Glandulars
	Raw/Whole? Frozen? Juiced? Smoothied?		Tea? Capsules? Raw/Whole? Dried?
05:00			
06:00			
07:00			
08:00			
09:00			
10:00			
11:00			
12:00			
13:00			
14:00			
15:00			
16:00			
17:00			
18:00			
19:00			
18:00			
19:00			
20:00			
21:00			
22:00			
23:00			

Slept or Fasted	Amount of Water Consumed	Sun Exposure	Lymph Exercises (E.g. Rebounder, Inversion, High Jumps, Sauna)

Date_________________________

Time	Fruits	Vegetables	Herbs/ Glandulars
	Raw/Whole? Frozen? Juiced? Smoothied?		Tea? Capsules? Raw/Whole? Dried?
05:00			
06:00			
07:00			
08:00			
09:00			
10:00			
11:00			
12:00			
13:00			
14:00			
15:00			
16:00			
17:00			
18:00			
19:00			
18:00			
19:00			
20:00			
21:00			
22:00			
23:00			

E.g. Rebounder, Inversion, High Jumps, Sauna

Slept or Fasted	Amount of Water Consumed	Sun Exposure	Lymph Exercises

Date______________________________

Time	Fruits	Vegetables	Herbs/ Glandulars
	Raw/Whole? Frozen? Juiced? Smoothied?		Tea? Capsules? Raw/Whole? Dried?
05:00			
06:00			
07:00			
08:00			
09:00			
10:00			
11:00			
12:00			
13:00			
14:00			
15:00			
16:00			
17:00			
18:00			
19:00			
18:00			
19:00			
20:00			
21:00			
22:00			
23:00			

E.g. Rebounder, Inversion, High Jumps, Sauna

Slept or Fasted	Amount of Water Consumed	Sun Exposure	Lymph Exercises

Date__________________________

Time	Fruits	Vegetables	Herbs/ Glandulars
	Raw/Whole? Frozen? Juiced? Smoothied?		Tea? Capsules? Raw/Whole? Dried?
05:00			
06:00			
07:00			
08:00			
09:00			
10:00			
11:00			
12:00			
13:00			
14:00			
15:00			
16:00			
17:00			
18:00			
19:00			
18:00			
19:00			
20:00			
21:00			
22:00			
23:00			

E.g. Rebounder, Inversion, High Jumps, Sauna

Slept or Fasted	Amount of Water Consumed	Sun Exposure	Lymph Exercises

Date______________________________

	Raw/Whole? Frozen? Juiced? Smoothied?		Tea? Capsules? Raw/Whole? Dried?
Time	**Fruits**	**Vegetables**	**Herbs/ Glandulars**
05:00			
06:00			
07:00			
08:00			
09:00			
10:00			
11:00			
12:00			
13:00			
14:00			
15:00			
16:00			
17:00			
18:00			
19:00			
18:00			
19:00			
20:00			
21:00			
22:00			
23:00			

Slept or Fasted	Amount of Water Consumed	Sun Exposure	Lymph Exercises E.g. Rebounder, Inversion, High Jumps, Sauna

Date____________________________

Time	Fruits	Vegetables	Herbs/ Glandulars
	Raw/Whole? Frozen? Juiced? Smoothied?		Tea? Capsules? Raw/Whole? Dried?
05:00			
06:00			
07:00			
08:00			
09:00			
10:00			
11:00			
12:00			
13:00			
14:00			
15:00			
16:00			
17:00			
18:00			
19:00			
18:00			
19:00			
20:00			
21:00			
22:00			
23:00			

E.g. Rebounder, Inversion, High Jumps, Sauna

Slept or Fasted	Amount of Water Consumed	Sun Exposure	Lymph Exercises

Date___________________________

Time	Fruits	Vegetables	Herbs/ Glandulars
	Raw/Whole? Frozen? Juiced? Smoothied?		Tea? Capsules? Raw/Whole? Dried?
05:00			
06:00			
07:00			
08:00			
09:00			
10:00			
11:00			
12:00			
13:00			
14:00			
15:00			
16:00			
17:00			
18:00			
19:00			
18:00			
19:00			
20:00			
21:00			
22:00			
23:00			

E.g.
Rebounder,
Inversion, High
Jumps, Sauna

Slept or Fasted	Amount of Water Consumed	Sun Exposure	Lymph Exercises

Date______________________________

	Raw/Whole? Frozen? Juiced? Smoothied?		Tea? Capsules? Raw/Whole? Dried?
Time	**Fruits**	**Vegetables**	**Herbs/ Glandulars**
05:00			
06:00			
07:00			
08:00			
09:00			
10:00			
11:00			
12:00			
13:00			
14:00			
15:00			
16:00			
17:00			
18:00			
19:00			
18:00			
19:00			
20:00			
21:00			
22:00			
23:00			

E.g. Rebounder, Inversion, High Jumps, Sauna

Slept or Fasted	Amount of Water Consumed	Sun Exposure	Lymph Exercises

Date______________________________

Time	Fruits	Vegetables	Herbs/ Glandulars
	Raw/Whole? Frozen? Juiced? Smoothied?		Tea? Capsules? Raw/Whole? Dried?
05:00			
06:00			
07:00			
08:00			
09:00			
10:00			
11:00			
12:00			
13:00			
14:00			
15:00			
16:00			
17:00			
18:00			
19:00			
18:00			
19:00			
20:00			
21:00			
22:00			
23:00			

E.g. Rebounder, Inversion, High Jumps, Sauna

Slept or Fasted	Amount of Water Consumed	Sun Exposure	Lymph Exercises

Date____________________________

	Raw/Whole? Frozen? Juiced? Smoothied?		Tea? Capsules? Raw/Whole? Dried?
Time	**Fruits**	**Vegetables**	**Herbs/ Glandulars**
05:00			
06:00			
07:00			
08:00			
09:00			
10:00			
11:00			
12:00			
13:00			
14:00			
15:00			
16:00			
17:00			
18:00			
19:00			
18:00			
19:00			
20:00			
21:00			
22:00			
23:00			

E.g. Rebounder, Inversion, High Jumps, Sauna

Slept or Fasted	Amount of Water Consumed	Sun Exposure	Lymph Exercises

Date____________________________

Time	Fruits	Vegetables	Herbs/ Glandulars
	Raw/Whole? Frozen? Juiced? Smoothied?		Tea? Capsules? Raw/Whole? Dried?
05:00			
06:00			
07:00			
08:00			
09:00			
10:00			
11:00			
12:00			
13:00			
14:00			
15:00			
16:00			
17:00			
18:00			
19:00			
18:00			
19:00			
20:00			
21:00			
22:00			
23:00			

E.g. Rebounder, Inversion, High Jumps, Sauna

Slept or Fasted	Amount of Water Consumed	Sun Exposure	Lymph Exercises

Date________________________

Time	Fruits	Vegetables	Herbs/ Glandulars
	Raw/Whole? Frozen? Juiced? Smoothied?		Tea? Capsules? Raw/Whole? Dried?
05:00			
06:00			
07:00			
08:00			
09:00			
10:00			
11:00			
12:00			
13:00			
14:00			
15:00			
16:00			
17:00			
18:00			
19:00			
18:00			
19:00			
20:00			
21:00			
22:00			
23:00			

E.g. Rebounder, Inversion, High Jumps, Sauna

Slept or Fasted	Amount of Water Consumed	Sun Exposure	Lymph Exercises

Date______________________________

Time	Fruits	Vegetables	Herbs/ Glandulars
	Raw/Whole? Frozen? Juiced? Smoothied?		Tea? Capsules? Raw/Whole? Dried?
05:00			
06:00			
07:00			
08:00			
09:00			
10:00			
11:00			
12:00			
13:00			
14:00			
15:00			
16:00			
17:00			
18:00			
19:00			
18:00			
19:00			
20:00			
21:00			
22:00			
23:00			

E.g. Rebounder, Inversion, High Jumps, Sauna

Slept or Fasted	Amount of Water Consumed	Sun Exposure	Lymph Exercises

Date__________________________

Time	Fruits	Vegetables	Herbs/ Glandulars
	Raw/Whole? Frozen? Juiced? Smoothied?		Tea? Capsules? Raw/Whole? Dried?
05:00			
06:00			
07:00			
08:00			
09:00			
10:00			
11:00			
12:00			
13:00			
14:00			
15:00			
16:00			
17:00			
18:00			
19:00			
18:00			
19:00			
20:00			
21:00			
22:00			
23:00			

E.g. Rebounder, Inversion, High Jumps, Sauna

Slept or Fasted	Amount of Water Consumed	Sun Exposure	Lymph Exercises

Date________________________

Time	Fruits	Vegetables	Herbs/ Glandulars
	Raw/Whole? Frozen? Juiced? Smoothied?		Tea? Capsules? Raw/Whole? Dried?
05:00			
06:00			
07:00			
08:00			
09:00			
10:00			
11:00			
12:00			
13:00			
14:00			
15:00			
16:00			
17:00			
18:00			
19:00			
18:00			
19:00			
20:00			
21:00			
22:00			
23:00			

E.g. Rebounder, Inversion, High Jumps, Sauna

Slept or Fasted	Amount of Water Consumed	Sun Exposure	Lymph Exercises

Date____________________________

Time	Fruits	Vegetables	Herbs/ Glandulars
	Raw/Whole? Frozen? Juiced? Smoothied?		Tea? Capsules? Raw/Whole? Dried?
05:00			
06:00			
07:00			
08:00			
09:00			
10:00			
11:00			
12:00			
13:00			
14:00			
15:00			
16:00			
17:00			
18:00			
19:00			
18:00			
19:00			
20:00			
21:00			
22:00			
23:00			

E.g. Rebounder, Inversion, High Jumps, Sauna

Slept or Fasted	Amount of Water Consumed	Sun Exposure	Lymph Exercises

Date______________________________

Time	Fruits	Vegetables	Herbs/ Glandulars
	Raw/Whole? Frozen? Juiced? Smoothied?		Tea? Capsules? Raw/Whole? Dried?
05:00			
06:00			
07:00			
08:00			
09:00			
10:00			
11:00			
12:00			
13:00			
14:00			
15:00			
16:00			
17:00			
18:00			
19:00			
18:00			
19:00			
20:00			
21:00			
22:00			
23:00			

E.g. Rebounder, Inversion, High Jumps, Sauna

Slept or Fasted	Amount of Water Consumed	Sun Exposure	Lymph Exercises

Date________________________

Time	Fruits	Vegetables	Herbs/ Glandulars
	Raw/Whole? Frozen? Juiced? Smoothied?		Tea? Capsules? Raw/Whole? Dried?
05:00			
06:00			
07:00			
08:00			
09:00			
10:00			
11:00			
12:00			
13:00			
14:00			
15:00			
16:00			
17:00			
18:00			
19:00			
18:00			
19:00			
20:00			
21:00			
22:00			
23:00			

Slept or Fasted	Amount of Water Consumed	Sun Exposure	E.g. Rebounder, Inversion, High Jumps, Sauna Lymph Exercises

Date________________________

Time	Fruits	Vegetables	Herbs/ Glandulars
	Raw/Whole? Frozen? Juiced? Smoothied?		Tea? Capsules? Raw/Whole? Dried?
05:00			
06:00			
07:00			
08:00			
09:00			
10:00			
11:00			
12:00			
13:00			
14:00			
15:00			
16:00			
17:00			
18:00			
19:00			
18:00			
19:00			
20:00			
21:00			
22:00			
23:00			

E.g. Rebounder, Inversion, High Jumps, Sauna

Slept or Fasted	Amount of Water Consumed	Sun Exposure	Lymph Exercises

Date________________________

Time	Fruits	Vegetables	Herbs/ Glandulars
	Raw/Whole? Frozen? Juiced? Smoothied?		Tea? Capsules? Raw/Whole? Dried?
05:00			
06:00			
07:00			
08:00			
09:00			
10:00			
11:00			
12:00			
13:00			
14:00			
15:00			
16:00			
17:00			
18:00			
19:00			
18:00			
19:00			
20:00			
21:00			
22:00			
23:00			

Slept or Fasted	Amount of Water Consumed	Sun Exposure	Lymph Exercises (E.g. Rebounder, Inversion, High Jumps, Sauna)

Date________________________

Time	Fruits	Vegetables	Herbs/ Glandulars
	Raw/Whole? Frozen? Juiced? Smoothied?		Tea? Capsules? Raw/Whole? Dried?
05:00			
06:00			
07:00			
08:00			
09:00			
10:00			
11:00			
12:00			
13:00			
14:00			
15:00			
16:00			
17:00			
18:00			
19:00			
18:00			
19:00			
20:00			
21:00			
22:00			
23:00			

E.g. Rebounder, Inversion, High Jumps, Sauna

Slept or Fasted	Amount of Water Consumed	Sun Exposure	Lymph Exercises

Date________________________

Time	Fruits	Vegetables	Herbs/ Glandulars
	Raw/Whole? Frozen? Juiced? Smoothied?		Tea? Capsules? Raw/Whole? Dried?
05:00			
06:00			
07:00			
08:00			
09:00			
10:00			
11:00			
12:00			
13:00			
14:00			
15:00			
16:00			
17:00			
18:00			
19:00			
18:00			
19:00			
20:00			
21:00			
22:00			
23:00			

Slept or Fasted	Amount of Water Consumed	Sun Exposure	Lymph Exercises (E.g. Rebounder, Inversion, High Jumps, Sauna)

Date______________________________

	Raw/Whole? Frozen? Juiced? Smoothied?		Tea? Capsules? Raw/Whole? Dried?
Time	**Fruits**	**Vegetables**	**Herbs/ Glandulars**
05:00			
06:00			
07:00			
08:00			
09:00			
10:00			
11:00			
12:00			
13:00			
14:00			
15:00			
16:00			
17:00			
18:00			
19:00			
18:00			
19:00			
20:00			
21:00			
22:00			
23:00			

E.g. Rebounder, Inversion, High Jumps, Sauna

Slept or Fasted	Amount of Water Consumed	Sun Exposure	Lymph Exercises

Date________________________

Time	Fruits	Vegetables	Herbs/ Glandulars
	Raw/Whole? Frozen? Juiced? Smoothied?		Tea? Capsules? Raw/Whole? Dried?
05:00			
06:00			
07:00			
08:00			
09:00			
10:00			
11:00			
12:00			
13:00			
14:00			
15:00			
16:00			
17:00			
18:00			
19:00			
18:00			
19:00			
20:00			
21:00			
22:00			
23:00			

E.g. Rebounder, Inversion, High Jumps, Sauna

Slept or Fasted	Amount of Water Consumed	Sun Exposure	Lymph Exercises

Date______________________________

Time	Fruits	Vegetables	Herbs/ Glandulars
	Raw/Whole? Frozen? Juiced? Smoothied?		Tea? Capsules? Raw/Whole? Dried?
05:00			
06:00			
07:00			
08:00			
09:00			
10:00			
11:00			
12:00			
13:00			
14:00			
15:00			
16:00			
17:00			
18:00			
19:00			
18:00			
19:00			
20:00			
21:00			
22:00			
23:00			

E.g. Rebounder, Inversion, High Jumps, Sauna

Slept or Fasted	Amount of Water Consumed	Sun Exposure	Lymph Exercises

Date______________________________

Time	Raw/Whole? Frozen? Juiced? Smoothied? Fruits	Vegetables	Tea? Capsules? Raw/Whole? Dried? Herbs/ Glandulars
05:00			
06:00			
07:00			
08:00			
09:00			
10:00			
11:00			
12:00			
13:00			
14:00			
15:00			
16:00			
17:00			
18:00			
19:00			
18:00			
19:00			
20:00			
21:00			
22:00			
23:00			

E.g.
Rebounder,
Inversion, High
Jumps, Sauna

Slept or Fasted	Amount of Water Consumed	Sun Exposure	Lymph Exercises

Date____________________

Time	Fruits	Vegetables	Herbs/ Glandulars
	Raw/Whole? Frozen? Juiced? Smoothied?		Tea? Capsules? Raw/Whole? Dried?
05:00			
06:00			
07:00			
08:00			
09:00			
10:00			
11:00			
12:00			
13:00			
14:00			
15:00			
16:00			
17:00			
18:00			
19:00			
18:00			
19:00			
20:00			
21:00			
22:00			
23:00			

E.g. Rebounder, Inversion, High Jumps, Sauna

Slept or Fasted	Amount of Water Consumed	Sun Exposure	Lymph Exercises

Date________________________

Time	Fruits	Vegetables	Herbs/ Glandulars
	Raw/Whole? Frozen? Juiced? Smoothied?		Tea? Capsules? Raw/Whole? Dried?
05:00			
06:00			
07:00			
08:00			
09:00			
10:00			
11:00			
12:00			
13:00			
14:00			
15:00			
16:00			
17:00			
18:00			
19:00			
18:00			
19:00			
20:00			
21:00			
22:00			
23:00			

Slept or Fasted	Amount of Water Consumed	Sun Exposure	Lymph Exercises (E.g. Rebounder, Inversion, High Jumps, Sauna)

Date________________________

Time	Fruits	Vegetables	Herbs/ Glandulars
	Raw/Whole? Frozen? Juiced? Smoothied?		Tea? Capsules? Raw/Whole? Dried?
05:00			
06:00			
07:00			
08:00			
09:00			
10:00			
11:00			
12:00			
13:00			
14:00			
15:00			
16:00			
17:00			
18:00			
19:00			
18:00			
19:00			
20:00			
21:00			
22:00			
23:00			

E.g. Rebounder, Inversion, High Jumps, Sauna

Slept or Fasted	Amount of Water Consumed	Sun Exposure	Lymph Exercises

Made in the USA
Las Vegas, NV
12 February 2022

43822107R00035